MW01289340

Sleep:
No More
Sleepless Nights

Overcome Insomnia, Increase Energy, Have Better

Health, and Get the Best Rest of Your Life!

By

Richard Wilson

Table of Contents

Introduction

I want to thank you and congratulate you for purchasing the book, Sleep: No More Sleepless Nights.

Everyone needs a good night's rest. A lot of people make the faulty assumption of sleep being some sort of downtime in the body, and that lack of sleep simply results in a drowsy day.

You may have stumbled upon this book for several reasons:

- You feel tired even after getting 8+ hours of sleep

- You can't seem to sleep right when you need to

- Your sleep keeps being interrupted and you don't know why

This book will help you solve most of the sleep problems people have through practical solutions. From the basics of sleep to more advanced treatment for sleep problems, we're going to have an all-out attack on what's preventing you from getting your well-deserved rest. This book will show you how deep sleep is achieved and what it achieves, so that you no longer have to drag yourself out of bed every morning or force yourself to count sheep at night.

Thanks again for purchasing this book, I hope you enjoy it!

CHAPTER 1

The Foundations of Sleep

It may not seem obvious, but what we do and what we aspire for are largely rooted in the amount of energy and type of mood we have, and those two aspects are usually inseparable. In most cases, you'd probably accept more difficult tasks and responsibilities when you're in a pretty good mood, and then after this good mood passes and you end up with zapped energy levels, you wonder why you've accepted this task in the first place.

That said, your body needs three main things to achieve stable energy levels and mood:

1. Food

2. Exercise

3. Sleep

Food provides your body with nutrients it needs to regenerate, repair, and recharge. Exercise places a good kind of stress on your system, therefore forcing your muscles to breakdown and rebuild stronger ones, while helping blood flow more efficiently to different parts of your body. Although some of the effects of food and exercise can be immediately felt, most of the important benefits they provide actually take place during sleep.

A lot of people try to live healthier lifestyles by going through absurd diets and hardcore exercises, only to find themselves still lethargic, sickly, and moody. Good quality sleep goes hand in hand with adequate nutrition and exercise; it helps you focus better and think more clearly, and it even makes you more sociable. On average, people need 7-9 hours of sleep every night to allow their bodies to recuperate, flush out stress, and consolidate fragments of ideas and memories.

Your body can recuperate when you're awake, but it can't do so as effectively as when you're asleep because it also has to distribute energy towards other bodily functions you may be using, like working, doing chores, catching up with a friend, etc. This is why bed rest is highly recommended for people who are sick; when you're asleep, your body can allocate significantly more energy towards healing. In a similar way, stress relief and memory consolidation are significantly more effectively done when you're asleep, as your brain isn't performing other thinking tasks.

The Stages of Sleep

There may be times when you've gotten 8-10 hours of sleep, only to find yourself groggy and tired throughout the day, but there also may be times when you've gotten only 5 hours of sleep or less but are zipping with energy from dawn to dusk. This is because the duration of sleep is only one part of the equation. In the same manner that eating a lot of junk food won't provide you with as much energy as eating moderate amounts of healthy food, getting lots of low quality sleep also won't provide you with nearly as much energy as getting low-moderate amounts of high quality sleep. This isn't to say, however, that quantity and quality don't go hand in hand; your body needs time to be able to start going into deep restorative sleep and also to be able to get out of that state.

If you've experienced completely draining your phone's battery, you'd notice that when you charge the phone, it needs a bit of time before you can turn it on and access its normal functions. This short period of time is like the phone's deep sleep mode; it needs a stable amount of energy provided without any other functions being accessed to regenerate enough power to "wake up".

Brainwaves tell us quite a lot about what happens when we sleep. Scientists have observed that sleep consists of several stages, going from a state of alert wakefulness to light stages of sleep, then to deep stages of sleep. This cycle is repeated a couple of times during a full night's rest. Here's a more thorough breakdown:

1. Non-REM (rapid eye movement) stage 1 – This state is rather volatile, as your body is actually half-awake and half-asleep. Even the subtlest sources of sound and light are enough to wake you up.

2. Non-REM stages 2-4 – If you don't wake up while going through stage 1, your sleep slowly reaches the stages 2-4. About 80% of sleep happens here.

3. REM – Finally, your body transitions into a short REM phase, which is what effectively restores and rejuvenates your energy. Dreaming means that you're going through this stage at least once. In this phase, your body is almost completely paralyzed to prevent you from acting out your dreams. The REM stage you experience in the first cycle of sleep is only about ten minutes, and as you experience more cycles of sleep, you experience longer REM stages, with 60 minutes being the theoretical maximum.

Typically, each cycle of sleep, from Non-REM stage 1 to REM, takes about 1.5 hours to happen, with about five cycles of sleep being more or less ideal. This is why you'd most likely hear people talking about getting 8 hours of sleep to feel refreshed in the morning; you'd have better chances of getting five cycles of sleep.

By understanding the basic stages of sleep, you can effectively plan when you need to go to sleep if you plan to wake up at a particular time. On average, it takes about 14 minutes to fall asleep, so if you need to wake up at 5:00 a.m., you can go to sleep at about 9:16 p.m. to get about five sleep cycles. This is, of course, assuming that you aren't interrupted during a sleep cycle. If you keep waking up every hour, your body may not experience REM sleep at all, and even 12 hours of sleep won't make you feel refreshed when you wake up. Remember, though, that even though five cycles of sleep is what most people need to feel refreshed in the morning, some people, because of their genetics, need either more or less sleep cycles to feel refreshed. Try out different numbers of sleep cycles to find out what works best for you.

What Happens When You Don't Get Enough Quality Sleep

Moodiness and lethargy are only two of the many symptoms you'd experience when you lack quality sleep. Here are a few other alarming things that happen to your mind and body when you don't get a good shut-eye every night:

- Chances of obesity drastically increase – The link between obesity and lack of sleep isn't just anecdotal. Studies have shown that when the body doesn't get the proper amount of quality sleep, it increases the release of ghrelin, which is a hormone that tells your body that you're hungry, while decreasing the release of leptin, which is a hormone that tells your body that you're full. In a nutshell, your body forces you to keep eating because it can't seem to get the energy it needs from your inadequate sleep.

- Risk of diabetes increases – Studies have shown that even just a week of sleep deprivation can lead to approximately 20% increase in insulin resistance. Insulin lets your body use the glucose you get from food for energy, and if your body becomes resistant to insulin, your blood sugar levels rise to dangerous levels, therefore increasing the risks of developing type-2 diabetes.

- Cognitive functions decline – This is one of the symptoms of inadequate sleep you're most likely familiar with. When you lack quality sleep, you tend to have difficulty focusing on a single task, remembering even the simplest details, and even performing mundane day-to-day tasks. Because your brain was not able to completely consolidate the fragments of ideas and memories you've had from yesterday, it carries the thought loads of both today and yesterday.

- Emotions run wild – Have you ever experienced an immense amount of anxiety over a huge decision, only to wake up the night after feeling calm and serene?

- Reaction time drastically decreases – This is one of the most dangerous immediate effects of lack of sleep for people who perform tasks that require quick responses. So far, about 20% of car crashes are caused by drowsy drivers who either fall asleep on the road or were not fast enough to stop the car when needed. Remember, the blood alcohol content for legally drunk drivers is about 0.07%, and driving while sleepy is like driving with about 0.08% blood alcohol content. The effect worsens when liquor and sleep deprivation is combined, as sleep deprivation boosts the effects of alcohol, leading to even worse reaction times and decreased alertness levels.

- Immune system becomes compromised – Studies have found that people who lack quality sleep prevent their immune systems from detecting and fighting off even the common cold. Abnormal immune responses like allergies also become more frequent and intense.

SLEEP AND REST

Unfortunately, it's not just enough to understand what can happen to you when you don't get quality sleep. It's also important to understand how the body recuperates when you start to sleep.

One thing that will surprise you is the amount of brain activity that takes place when you sleep. Upon reaching the deeper levels of REM sleep, your brain starts to pick up just as much as it would if you were awake!

Since you no longer need to watch yourself breath and perform other daily activities, the brain takes this chance to do a lot of work in preparation for when you wake up.

Hormone Secretion

As surprising as this may sound, your body continuously makes growth hormones as you sleep; provided that you've entered the proper sleep cycle.

Unfortunately, these aren't the hormones that are supposed to make you grow taller. These are hormones meant to repair tissues that have been damaged during the day. This is because your body works on the healing process when you rest. There's no better time to focus on the body than when the owner is unconscious and immobilized.

Depending on your diet, your body may or may not make short work of your wounds. Healing also depends on the kind of damage the body needs to heal. Cuts and bruises usually take a few days. They become weeks without proper sleep patterns.

This is the reason why body builders prioritize sleeping and resting just as much as their trips to the gym. When they're awake, they tear their muscle tissue by lifting weights and doing all sorts of repetitions. When they sleep, their bodies repair their damaged muscle tissues and build better ones, toning and sculpting their bodies in the process.

Brain Connections

You might have already heard that sleeping well after a hard night of studying is one of the best ways to prepare for an exam. There's a science behind that.

On top of repairing damaged muscle tissues, the brain also establishes new neuron connections. That makes it easier for you to recall things in the morning. Couple that with a good rest and an alert state of mind, recalling important information become easier.

Surprisingly, the brain also dissolves unused connections that weren't used that much during the day. What you worried about during the day stays and becomes a permanent part of your consciousness. This contributes to chronic stress if all you do is worry. This will be discussed in a later chapter.

Temperature Drops

Besides repairs and optimizations, your core temperature begins to drop when you're asleep. As you already know, heat is generated by the body when you burn calories and engage in your daily activities. Since you're not engaged in anything physical other than breathing, your body has the chance to lower its temperature to allow other healing processes to take place.

Remember that for all these positive things to take place in the body, you have to be in a deep enough sleep cycle so that your body can kick it into high gear.

The Battle Plan

After getting an overview of sleep, its stages, and the types of problems lack of quality sleep can bring, the next step is to reexamine your day-to-day activities to discover what's keeping you from getting enough quality sleep. In the next chapter, we're going to talk about the best ways to "set the stage" for a restorative sleep. By doing so, you'll discover a lot of bad habits in your life that you need to get rid of to make way for good habits that help you reap the maximum benefits quality sleep could give you.

CHAPTER 2

Creating the Perfect Environment for Sleep

T his chapter consists of the first part of your sleep battle plan: setting the right mindset and context for quality sleep. The main focus of this chapter is to help you create an environment conducive to sleep so that your brain knows when it should be preparing your body to sleep and when it should be preparing your body to wake up.

Setting the Right Mindset

After several nights of restless sleep, it might seem impossible to change habits that you're already used to. Adaptation requires your body to spend more energy than it's used to, but remember why you've started doing this, and what would happen if you stop. It takes approximately 21 days to build a habit, and if you vigilantly fight to get rid of bad habits and beliefs that keep you from getting quality sleep, after the 21 habit-building days, you're stuck with good habits that will stay with you for the rest of your life (or at least until you find a better habit to replace it with).

Creating an Environment Conducive to Sleep

Our minds are highly dependent on context. You may be familiar with this type of situation: you go into your bedroom, and all of a sudden, you feel thirsty. You go downstairs to the kitchen, but then you forget why you went to the kitchen in the first place. You go back up to your room, and then you suddenly remembered again that you were thirsty. That being said, your bedroom needs to be able to send your brain a message that it needs to sleep at night and wake up in the morning.

The brain performs tasks extremely well if they're done in consistent contexts. This is why offices have harsh, intense lighting and hotels have warm, subdued lighting; the brain becomes wide-awake and alert in brighter, whiter lights and relaxed and calm in warmer, yellowish lights.

Now that you know how important it is to set the right context for sleep, let's talk about how you can make your bedroom highly conducive to sleep.

Lighting: We've talked about office buildings having a whiter color than hotels, because the color temperature of lights greatly affect the REM sleep one gets. Any light source with a rating of about 6000k and above are considered cool, while any light source with a rating way below 6000k, usually 3000k, are considered warm.

In the times when we did not have artificial sources of light, our bodies were used to doing all the necessary activities during the day, and then winding down as the night approaches, finally sinking into a blissful sleep. Until now, our brains are wired to see daylight as a signal to stay awake and alert and the afternoon sunset as signals to calm down and rest. Daylight has a color temperature of approximately 6500k, slowly progressing into 3000k. Fluorescent lights typically used in the household have 6500k color temperatures, designed to keep everyone wide awake until they're turned off. Our gadgets emit blue lights, which further boost alertness and wakefulness – good for the day, but bad for the night.

That said, here are guidelines you'll want to follow to prevent light from interfering with your sleep:

- Total Darkness is Best - Whenever possible, opt for a pitch-black environment for sleeping. This makes it easier for your mind to fall asleep because it won't be distracted by things in your bedroom. Also, being enclosed in total darkness lets your pineal gland produce melatonin, which is what gets your mind into the REM state.

- Avoid Bright Lights 2-3 Hours before Bedtime – You don't need your bedroom to be as dark as a cave when you're getting ready to sleep, you just need to avoid bright sources of light 2-3 hours before bedtime. Bright lights can confuse your brain by making it think that it's only 3:00 pm in the afternoon when it's actually 1:00 am in the morning. You'll still be able to fall asleep, but the type of sleep your body will give you is the shallow afternoon slumber that isn't as restorative as a full night's sleep.

- Use Gadgets with Smaller Screens – Blue light is effective in suppressing melatonin. Naturally, that'd mean that gadgets with larger screens emit more of this blue light. Whenever you can, go for gadgets with smaller screens.

- Use Adaptive Display-Altering Apps – If you find yourself needing to use laptops and other devices with large screens late at night, you can use apps like F.lux that automatically changes the color of your screen based on the time of day. Basically, these types of apps make your screen look rather yellow or orange, effectively filtering out more of the harmful blue or green wavelengths and therefore making less of an impact on your sleep. Some devices, however, may not allow changes to screen color on a software level, so instead, you can opt for physical filters that remove blue wavelengths from any source of light. Orange filter theatrical gels are reportedly effective at doing this.

- Red Light > Blue Light – Notice how darkrooms have only red lights to prevent photos from getting ruined? If you can't seem to fall asleep in full darkness, the next best thing is getting a red night lamp, as it has been proven to provide the least disturbance in terms of REM sleep. Blue lights are out of the question, as they basically tell your brain to wake up by suppressing melatonin.

- Go Out and Experience the Sun! – Strangely, people who are exposed to daylight longer have fewer problems getting a good night's sleep. Sunlight strongly affects your circadian rhythm, which is basically your inner clock that tells you when to sleep and when to wake up. Expose yourself to more sunlight by taking walks a few times a day outside, and you'll notice yourself sleeping more soundly.

Sound: No matter how dark your room is, if neighborhood dogs decide to form an all-night ensemble, you're going to end up being their involuntary audience. Here are some options for you to consider:

- Get Rid of the Sound Source – This is the most obvious and simplest solution to the noise problems you may be encountering, though it may not be possible in some cases, like if you live in a busy street with irregular beeps, honks, and screeches. In the case of dripping faucets and other things that you have control over, though, it follows that this should be your first option.

- Use Ear Plugs – Although your body may not be used to sleeping in complete silence, it'll definitely adapt better compared to the irregular sounds produced by urban surroundings. Studies have shown that sounds produced by stereos, televisions, and other gadgets are almost always "noisier" than nature, regardless of their volume. This is why, in heavily populated cities, you'd seldom hear birds chirping or leaves rustling. The only downside to this is that you won't be able to hear your alarm if you're using one.

- Listen to Repetitive Instrumentals – Don't want to sleep in total silence? You can listen to a few repetitive instrumentals that don't evoke emotions or provoke analytical thinking. In the past, cavemen had to quickly awaken when they hear a predator approaching or a tribe member crying for help. Until now, our brains are still wired to scan for any abrupt changes in sound that might be dangerous. This is why you don't want music with varying intensity blasted in your ears when you're sleeping; an abrupt transition from the verse to chorus is enough to pull you out of REM sleep.

- Try Out Binaural Beats – Binaural beats straddle the line between medical science and "quack" science. Researchers are still debating whether or not the science behind binaural beats is sound. Nevertheless, a lot of people have reported having better quality sleep after listening to binaural beats overnight, so you'll need to try them out for yourself and see if they truly are effective.

There are basically four brainwave frequencies that dictate our mental and physical state:

- Beta (13-40 Hz) – Alert, awake, and focused

- Alpha (8-12 Hz) – Calm, creative, and relaxed

- Theta (4-8 Hz) – Very sleepy or in a state of light sleep

- Delta (< 4 Hz) – Deep sleep (REM)

The ideal transition of your brain's states is from the beta state, which is usually when you do tasks that require strong analytical skills or physical strength, to the alpha state, which is usually when you're done with the day's activities and are now winding down, reading a good book, writing a blog entry, etc., to the theta state, which is usually when you're already in bed trying to sleep or are already lightly sleeping, to the delta state, which is where the elusive REM sleep resides. As you see, the process in going to the delta state can be quite long, which is why people resort to using binaural beats.

You'll need to use earbuds, because binaural beats emit sound waves with different frequencies in each earbud, therefore forcing your brain to somehow follow that difference in frequency. For example, playing sound waves with 440 Hz in one ear and 448 Hz will result in your brain supposedly being forced into a theta state. Pure binaural beats will sound like monotonous hums, which is why some of the ones available online are combined with background audio. You'll want to go for the pure ones for maximum effectiveness.

- Use Gentler Alarm Clock Sounds – Whenever your loud, harsh alarm goes off, your body produces a surge of adrenaline. Unfortunately, if you keep waking up like this, your adrenal glands will get tired, and you begin to feel less of the effects of adrenalin when you actually need it. Loud, harsh alarm sounds also make mornings more unbearable as it yanks you out of dream world in a split second. You'll want to try something that can wake you up using soothing music that gradually increases in volume. You can combine this with a wake-up light that simulates the rising sun by increasing its intensity gradually along with its color temperature.

Temperature: Cooler temperatures are best for falling asleep, as the night is often cooler than the day, and our brains are wired to fall asleep when the core body temperature drops. If your room is warm, your body may find it too uncomfortable to fall asleep and stay asleep, therefore giving you interrupted bits of sleep that isn't restorative or deep. A temperature of about 68 degrees Fahrenheit is recommended, with 75 degrees Fahrenheit as the upper limit and 54 degrees Fahrenheit as the lower limit.

Here are some ways to help you keep your body and your room temperature stable and conducive to sleep:

- DIY Air Conditioner – Not everyone can afford air conditioners and the electricity bill hikes they cause. Fortunately, you can create a DIY air conditioner that fits your budget and your environment. The simplest type of DIY air conditioner is a regular electric fan with a shallow bowl filled with ice placed in front of it. The fan basically blows the ice, causing it to melt and evaporate, therefore effectively reducing the ambient temperature.

- Get a Cooling Pillow – Sometimes, the reason you flip and turn through the night is that your pillow gets too warm for your head. Cooling pillows help keep your head cool, therefore effectively helping you sleep throughout the night uninterrupted. In addition to the uninterrupted sleep, studies show that the brain performs memory consolidation and other important tasks better when it's operating at relatively cool temperatures, which means that with a cooling pillow, you may actually think more clearly when you wake up because your brain was able to perform more tasks when you were asleep.

- Refrigerate Your Sheets – Technically, this won't help you sleep through a ridiculously hot night, but it will definitely help you fall asleep faster if the temperature isn't too bad. You'll want to put your sheets in a sealed plastic bag and put them in your refrigerator for a few minutes, making sure that no moisture gets in the sheets. When you're ready to sleep, simply put the cooled sheets in bed and quickly get in, as your body will quickly warm the sheets. The cooled sheets should help you fall asleep quickly, but in the case of extremely hot temperatures, it will do very little to help you stay asleep.

- Dampen Your Sheets – This method works better than refrigerating your sheets, as it lasts longer, but it can be a hassle to do every night. You basically soak your sheets in cold water, and then wring them out until they are only damp but not soaking wet. When you use this as a blanket, evaporative cooling will take place and when you wake up, your blanket should be completely dry and you should be completely refreshed. If you don't find yourself comfortable sleeping in damp sheets, you can opt for smaller variations, like damp, cool washcloths on your head or damp, cool socks on your feet.

- Generate Cool Breeze – If you'd rather not get any part of your body wet with cold water when you sleep, you can simply place damp sheets in front of an open window. Evaporative cooling should also take place and reduce the ambient room temperature enough to help you fall asleep. In hotter climates, however, this method may be too short-lived to be of any use.

- Dampen Your Hair – If you don't mind your hair getting a bit frizzy and messed-up in the morning, sleeping with damp hair will help keep your head cooler in the night through evaporative cooling.

- Sleep in the Basement – The basement is often significantly cooler than the rest of the house because it's well insulated. When heat waves attack, you can simply opt to sleep in the basement for a few days until the temperature in your room becomes bearable again.

- Stay in a Low Position – Can't or don't want to sleep in the basement? You may just need to sleep at a lower level in your room, whether that means getting a bed with shorter legs or moving your mattress to the floor. Because heat rises, you'll feel a lot cooler in the lower parts of your room.

Mattress and Pillows: A comfortable mattress and the right pillows make sure that your body remains comfortable enough to stay asleep the whole night.

To get the right pillow, you'll have to take your sleeping style into consideration. A general guideline for picking a pillow is that it has to keep your head and neck aligned as if you were standing up. Here are more specific guidelines for choosing the right pillow depending on your sleeping style:

- Sleeping on your stomach – This type of sleeping generally isn't recommended, as it often leads to neck pain and problems with your lower back. You'll want to change this sleeping style by attaching something uncomfortable (a Lego, maybe?) to your stomach so that when you flip to this sleeping position, the object attached to your stomach will wake you up and force you to change positions. This'll initially disrupt your sleep, but in the long run, it'll lead to better quality sleep and less back and neck pains.

- Sleeping on your side – You'll want to get a pillow to help prevent your head from becoming misaligned with your neck when you lie down. A pillow between your knees also helps align your spine better because your feet won't curve or bend in an unnatural way.

- Sleeping on your back – Sleeping on your back is reportedly the best sleeping position to date. You'll want to invest in a memory foam, as it adapts to the natural curve of your neck and therefore prevents neck pains.

It can be quite difficult to shop for a low-priced, quality mattress because mattress makers tend to give the same products different names specifically so that customers wouldn't be able to compare prices easily. This basically means that you can't buy mattresses based on how they're named or wrapped. That said, it's best to purchase mattresses that have a good return policy so that you can try out mattresses that are fairly priced and work your way up if the current mattress doesn't work for you. In general, however, here are the most common types of mattresses you can choose from:

- Sleep Number Beds – Sleep number beds actually have customizable levels of firmness. Although sleep number beds are often pricier than regular mattresses, they're great investments for people who want to try out different levels of firmness or couples who have different preferences in terms of firmness (because some sleep number beds have different chambers that allow different firmness levels on different sides of the bed).

- Memory Foam Beds – Some mattresses use memory foams that basically adapt to your body shape as you sleep to provide even support. Take note that while these types of mattresses are said to be very comfortable and even therapeutic, they tend to get warmer throughout the night compared to other mattresses. If you don't have an air conditioning system, this type of mattress may not be for you.

- Permanently Firm Beds – Firm mattresses are often preferred, as they don't allow your body to curve in an unhealthy manner. If you're used to sleeping in plush mattresses, however, it may take a few days or weeks to fall asleep soundly on a firm mattress.

- Permanently Plushy Beds – A lot of people like plushy beds especially when used in an air-conditioned room. Take note, however, that these types of mattresses typically cause back and neck pains because of their lack of support. In rooms without air conditioning, plushy beds tend to further contain heat, causing your body to overheat and force you to wake up. In most cases, you're better off investing in firm memory foam beds.

Bedroom Color: The colors present in your room can significantly affect how well you sleep at night. To date, here are the three best colors in promoting sleep:

- Pale Blue – The state associated with the color blue is calmness and security. This is why a lot of social media sites and banks use this color in their logos and interfaces. In the bedroom, a paler shade of blue is said to promote calmness that helps people fall asleep faster.

- Pale Yellow – Yellow is another color known for promoting calmness and relaxation, however, it may make a room too bright if other shades of this color are chosen.

- Green – Green in any shade is said to be easier on the eyes, which is why it's an ideal color for people who also have to work in their bedrooms. What's great about this color is that it takes a bit longer before your eyes get tired when you're working, but it also relaxes them enough to let you sleep. People who have green bedrooms also report waking up more alert and refreshed.

CHAPTER 3

Sleep Habits Do's and Don'ts

So far, we've talked about ways to make your bedroom more conducive to sleep. Now it's time to fine-tune your habits, getting rid of ones that hinder sleep to make way for ones that promote sleep. Along with context, the mind likes routine. Your brain actually rewires itself to be more efficient in doing tasks it knows it's going to do regularly.

Before talking about habits that promote sleep, let's talk about habits that hinder sleep and what you can do about them:

Caffeine before Bed: The primary purpose of caffeine is to prevent sleep. The half-life of caffeine is about 6 hours, which means that if you drink a cup of coffee at 1 pm, you'll end up with half a cup of coffee in your system at 7 pm. Even though some people argue that they could still fall asleep after drinking caffeine, caffeine actually lengthens the theta state while shortening the vital delta state. This is great for power naps, which shall be discussed later, but bad for a night's worth of rest. This means that although you may be able to fall asleep even as you drink a cup of coffee before bed, you may feel lightheaded in the morning because of the lack of restorative sleep. So far, studies have shown that abstinence from caffeine 6 hours before bedtime is best. If you find yourself still not having restful sleep, push back the caffeine time a bit more.

Alcohol before Bed: Some people consume alcohol before going to bed because it relaxes them enough to help them sleep. However, the danger in consuming alcohol before sleeping is that it wreaks havoc on your sleep cycles, causing you to wake up abruptly throughout the night. On average, it takes about 3 hours for the body to break down alcohol, so you'll want to stop consuming alcohol at least 3 hours before going to bed.

Heavy Meals before Bed: Ever heard of the rule "Eat breakfast like a king, lunch like a prince, and dinner like a pauper?" Your body needs to allocate as much energy as it can in healing, memory consolidation, and other tasks your brain normally wouldn't be able to do full-time when you're awake. If you eat too much carbs and hard-to-digest food like beef, your body will have to redirect more energy into your digestive system, therefore requiring more hours of sleep. The best type of dinner you can eat is one with fruits, veggies, and fish, as they're easier to break down and also provide more nutrients for your body to use when you're asleep. Some people have reported needing only about 5-6 hours of sleep when they have a light, pescetarian dinner, whereas people who have heavy, carb-loaded, meat-stuffed dinners tend to need 7-10 hours of sleep.

Going to Bed Hungry: Just because you want your body to focus on healing and energy regeneration doesn't mean that you should go to bed hungry. The key is to eat at least 2-4 hours before sleeping, with fewer hours needed for lighter meals and more hours for heavier meals. If you go to bed hungry, chances are, your stomach is going to wake you up for a midnight snack, therefore further throwing off your sleep cycle.

Going to Bed Thirsty: Your body, specifically your brain, needs at least 2 liters of water each day, more if you sweat a lot or are more active. If you want a more accurate gauge on how much water you need, studies show that for every 50 pounds of body weight, you'd need 1 quart of water. Going to bed thirsty has been observed to produce effects similar to sleep apnea. If you dislike the idea of drinking a glass of water before going to bed because it wakes you up at night, you can opt to drink water 2-4 hours before going to bed. A good indicator for hydration is your urine; if your urine is clear or a very pale yellow, then that means you're getting enough water.

Bad Sleeping Positions: If you tend to have muscle aches, snoring problems, or indigestion, a simple change in your sleeping position could be the key to curing all of those problems. Here are common problems you may experience after sleeping and their corresponding position-corrections:

- Neck ache – Neck aches are one of the most common problems people with bad sleeping positions have. In most cases, sleeping on the stomach or sleeping with too many pillows causes the neck to bend at unnatural angles. If you experience neck aches quite a lot, you'll need to keep your neck at a neutral position. Keep your pillow above your shoulders and perhaps use a rolled-up hand towel to support your neck so that its position remains neutral.

- Backache – Back pains are often caused by the fetal sleeping position. Remember that only unborn babies and people suffering from lumbar spinal stenosis are allowed to do a fetal sleeping position. For adults, this position places unneeded stress on your spine. Strive to sleep on your back while placing a pillow under your knees and a rolled hand towel under your lower back to help your spine align itself naturally.

  If you don't like sleeping on your back, you can sleep on your side instead, with a pillow between your knees to maintain a neutral position.

- Snoring – Although sleeping on your back is often the best sleeping position, for people with sleep apnea/snoring problems, this can actually impair breathing. You'll want to sleep on your side instead, while taping or sewing something uncomfortable on your back to prevent you from rolling onto your back.

- Acid reflux – You can either opt to sleep on your side or raise the head of your bed by placing stable material under the legs near the top, where you rest your head. Avoid trying to add more pillows, though, as this may cause a neck ache.

Working, Eating, etc., in Your Bedroom: As mentioned before, your brain performs tasks better when done in the right context. This is why you'd find it hard to eat in a bathroom or study in an amusement park. When you work inside your bedroom, two things can happen: you'd easily get drowsy while you work or you'd be alert and awake even when you try to sleep. Eating in your bedroom also may produce similar effects: you'd get drowsy as you eat (which isn't too bad), or you'd get hungry as soon as you try to sleep (this is bad). If eating or working in your bedroom is unavoidable, you'll want to make the context of eating or working clearly separate from sleeping, e.g., you'd have strong, brighter lights as you work, subdued, lights as you eat, and complete darkness as you sleep.

Oversleeping: A lot of people think that when they've missed a couple of hours of sleep in the week, oversleeping in the weekend can make up for it. However, remember that your body optimizes internal operations according to what's being done to it on a regular basis. This means that if you sleep in on weekends, you're going to find it hard to wake up early on weekdays again, throwing off your schedule and therefore causing you to lose more sleep. The key here is consistency; make sure that you wake up at the same time every day, taking power naps throughout the day to help you get some extra sleep without ruining your sleep schedule.

Snoozing the Alarm Clock: It may seem like you're doing your body a favor by sleeping for an extra 10 minutes, six to ten times before you actually get up, but you're actually depriving yourself of quality sleep. When you wake up, your body is already starting to transition into the alpha or beta state, causing alertness and wakefulness to start seeping into your brain. When you hit that snooze button and sleep for a few minutes, your brain stops the current transition and immediately tries to start another sleep cycle. However, as you enter another sleep cycle, the alarm clock wakes you up, causing an abrupt change in brainwave state. This makes you feel even worse as you keep hitting that snooze button. This habit is one of the hardest one to kick, as getting even just a few minutes of dreamland can feel like heaven, especially on Mondays. You'll have to set your alarm clock to the actual time you want to get up. Remember the tip about a slowly intensifying alarm and a slow-rise light? That tip should help your body transition into a more alert and wakeful state faster so that you won't have a chance to drift off into dreamland again.

Now that you know some of the worst habits that adversely affect sleep, here are some of the best ways you can promote sleep:

Exercise: Even with the most conducive sleeping environment, if your body isn't tired, it simply won't allow you to fall asleep. At least an hour's worth of physical activity with exposure to sunlight is critical in regulating your sleep cycle. When your body sees the change in context, from bright sunlight and plenty of physical movement to complete darkness and stillness, you'll find yourself falling asleep the moment your body hits the mattress.

Master the Art of Napping: Whether it takes you half an hour to sleep or just a few seconds, anyone can master the art of napping. A lot of people get napping and sleeping confused, as these two activities involve relaxing and closing one's eyes. However, in taking a nap, you actually don't need to fall asleep. You can simply relax, let your thoughts wander like a cloud, and not stress about not being able to fall asleep. A well-executed power nap can bring you from a state of mental exhaustion into a fresh, alert, and focused mind in 20 minutes. Here are simple steps you can follow to get a refreshing power nap:

1. Lie or sit down

2. Relax your body from head to toe

3. Let your thoughts drift away. Don't focus on any thought that comes to you.

4. Make a bit of effort to think about relaxing sceneries instead of stressful and embarrassing memories.

5. Keep your body relaxed, your eyes closed, and your thoughts floating blissfully.

6. After 20 minutes, get up. You may feel drowsy for a few minutes, but don't stay down; the drowsiness should be gone in a minute or two.

That's it! Napping doesn't actually need you to fall asleep to experience its amazing benefits. You're not reaching for REM sleep. Rather, you're reaching for theta sleep, which is a state of relaxation that straddles between the dream world and the real world. Remember not to go over the 20-minute limit. If you add an extra 10 minutes, your mind may start thinking that you're really trying to sleep and will start a complete sleep cycle. You're not going to enjoy waking up in the middle of this sleep cycle.

In most cases, napping is a better option than drinking a caffeinated drink. Unlike caffeine, your body won't build tolerance to naps, so you can take it a couple of times a day without losing its energizing effects. In cases where you lack sleep and really need your caffeine fix, however, you may opt to combine napping and caffeine. Your body needs about 14 minutes to fully absorb caffeine, so if you drink coffee before taking a nap, you should automatically wake up between 14-20 minutes, assuming that your body isn't too tolerant of caffeine.

Proper Supplementation: If you need to fall asleep faster, there are plenty of supplements that could knock you out in a couple of minutes, without leaving you groggy in the morning. Some of these supplements are also known to help you reach the delta state faster:

- Melatonin – Melatonin is a strong hormone and powerful antioxidant that your pineal gland produces to get you to the delta state. Your pineal gland starts producing melatonin in the right context (enough exercise, right amount of light, etc.). If you don't sleep well at night, chances are, you're not getting enough melatonin. There's been a lot of debate as to whether or not you should take melatonin supplements regularly because of the possibility of further suppressing your body's natural melatonin production. However, if you work in changing shifts or are experiencing jetlag, taking melatonin for a night or two will help you reset your biological clock. Go for the lowest dosage available (3 mg).

- GABA – GABA is one of the most powerful calming supplements available. You can use this during the day if you find yourself overwhelmed by stress, but in most cases, this works best if taken at night, as your brain actually uses needs this to transition from an alert (and perhaps stressed) state into deep sleep. You'll want to start with a 500 mg dosage and work your way up as you deem necessary to a maximum of 750 mg. For general stress relief, 250 mg is usually enough.

- L-tryptophan – Tryptophan is an important amino acid, but your body doesn't produce it, which is why you have to get it from foods like milk, turkey, and certain types of food and food supplements. The reason a lot of people advise drinking warm milk before going to bed is because of the small amounts of L-tryptophan it contains. Unfortunately, this amount of L-tryptophan is actually deemed ineffective in helping one sleep better; as it turns out, it's because of the warmness of the beverage that people are able to sleep better. Typically, 1-2 grams of L-tryptophan taken about 30 minutes before going to bed is enough to help you fall asleep. You'll want to start with 1 gram, adding 500 mg each night up to 3 grams, or until you're satisfied with the results it brings, whichever comes first.

- Chamomile tea – Chamomile tea is one of the most popular sleep-inducing herbs. It's known to have anti-anxiety effects, though there isn't enough conclusive evidence to support this. Some researchers have observed that the calming and soothing effects of chamomile tea actually come with any warm beverage and aren't actually caused by any ingredients exclusive to chamomile. A lot of people swear by its effects, though, so you'll want to try it for yourself and see if it helps you fall asleep faster.

- L-theanine – L-theanine is a popular partner of coffee, as it counteracts the jitters caused by the caffeine. 100 mg of L-theanine in capsule form is known to help you maintain a calm, focused state when working, especially under the influence of caffeine, but it can also prevent caffeine from jolting you out of REM sleep.

- Potassium and Magnesium – Potassium and magnesium are known to work especially well together in removing leg cramps that quickly yank people out of REM sleep. It's best to try both of these supplements on the low end, progressively going up if you feel you need more. For potassium, you'll want to find the citrate or bicarbonate forms, starting with 100 mg, with a maximum of 400 mg at bedtime. For magnesium, you'll want to start at 400 mg, with a maximum of 800 mg.

- Ornithine – Ornithine is a type of amino acid that relaxes your body by helping it get rid of excess ammonia in your stomach. Ammonia is acceptable in minute amounts, however, in excess, it causes stress and can also interfere with growth hormone production. Start with 1 gram and work your way up to 5 grams as you feel necessary.

- GHB – GHB currently has a bad reputation as a result of it being used as a date-rape drug. However, GHB is actually a medical drug approved by the U.S. Food and Drug Administration that is used to treat narcolepsy, which is a disorder that causes irregular sleep cycles and all-day lethargy. GHB is known to normalize sleep patterns effectively, causing a longer period of REM sleep while being almost completely gone from your system after just about 6 hours. In this list of supplements, GHB is probably the most powerful drug and has the most potential in helping you sleep deeply and wake up with overflowing energy. GHB is also non-addictive and will not interfere with your body's natural melatonin production. However, take note that GHB is a prescription drug and can be lethal when abused. You'll need to ask your doctor first before trying out this drug.

Eating "Sleepy Foods": Carbohydrate foods that have high glycemic rankings are known to help reduce the time it takes for people to fall asleep. Ever experience a sugar crash after eating a slice of cake or a doughnut? That's what we're somewhat aiming for in this list. You'll have to take these "sleepy foods" within 4 hours of bedtime to help your body release tryptophan and serotonin more quickly, as these chemicals induce restful sleep:

- Bread – French bread and plain bagels are great choices, as they both have high glycemic ranking but aren't too unhealthy to consume either.

- Cereal – Combine this with warm milk for a synergistic calming effect that'll surely help you fall asleep quickly.

- Potatoes – A lot of people report feeling sleepy after consuming potatoes, whether it's French fries or mashed potatoes. Avoid consuming oily ones, though, as it may end up upsetting your stomach.

- Sweets – You really shouldn't eat sweets like ice cream or doughnuts before going to bed, however, lighter form of sweets like graham crackers are acceptable and are even beneficial for a good night's rest.

- Watermelon – Watermelon is natural, and it helps rehydrate your body so that you don't wake up in the middle of the night parched.

- Honey – A lot of medical students have consumed pure honey for blood sugar experiments, only to find themselves extremely drowsy after a single teaspoon. If you're not comfortable taking a teaspoon of pure honey, you can combine it with warm milk or chamomile tea.

Eating Healthy Foods: Sugar crashes provide an almost immediate knockout, however, for people with strict diets and healthier lifestyles, a lot of the foods in the "sleepy foods" list may not be viable. That said, here are healthy foods that will help you fall asleep without ruining your diet:

- Bananas – Bananas should be in your weekly grocery list, as they are an abundant source of potassium and magnesium, which, as we talked about earlier, are good at relieving cramps by acting as natural muscle relaxants. Bananas also contain tryptophan, which is also a sleep-inducing amino acid, as we've discussed earlier. Two supplements in a single fruit is nothing to sneeze at, so make sure you have plenty of bananas in stock.

- Cherries – Cherries are one of the only natural sources of melatonin. Melatonin tablets contain way more melatonin than the body needs, which is why it can actually suppress the body's natural melatonin production. However, cherries contain safe amounts of melatonin, making them great choices for bedtime snacks or drinks.

- Oatmeal – A bowl of oatmeal actually provides magnesium, potassium, phosphorus, silicon, and calcium, which are all important nutrients that promote sleep. Unfortunately, however, most types of oatmeal don't particularly taste good without a lot of sugar. Because too much sugar will prevent you from having uninterrupted sleep, you'll want to go with a teaspoon of honey instead. This will result in possibly less flavorful oatmeal, but coupled with cherries and perhaps a banana, you have a tasty, wonderful, sleep-inducing meal.

- Decaf Green Tea – As mentioned before, L-theanine helps promote sleep. Green tea provides a good amount of L-theanine, but you'll have to make sure that the one you get doesn't have caffeine, otherwise, it defeats the purpose.

- High-protein foods – High-protein foods are known to promote sleep, while preventing heartburn from flaring up in the middle of the night and cutting your sleep short. You can eat something as simple as a hardboiled egg or cottage cheese with fruits that aren't too high in sugar.

- Milk – As mentioned before, milk contains small amounts of tryptophan (though reportedly not enough to be effective on its own), but it also contains calcium, which helps your body produce the right amount of melatonin. You can add a teaspoon of honey if you don't have problems with your blood sugar.

- Almonds – Almonds are full of protein, as well as magnesium. This means that consuming almonds before sleeping will help promote sleep as well as relax your muscles to prevent cramps from interrupting your sleep. You can try switching your regular milk to almond milk if you haven't already tried, as almond milk contains more protein than regular milk and is said to be a lot healthier.

CHAPTER 4

Sleep Hacks

This section contains a compilation of interesting methods for falling asleep that have worked for quite a lot of people. Some of these methods haven't been scientifically proven but seem to be quite effective, whether as a placebo effect or a true therapeutic effect. Some of these methods, on the other hand, don't directly affect sleep, but do help remove activities that do affect sleep. Nevertheless, these methods are safe to try and can be discarded if you don't see any positive changes in your sleep patterns:

- **Use Reverse Psychology on Yourself**: The University of Glasgow did a study with two different groups of insomniacs and observed how their sleep patterns changed throughout the experiment. One of the groups were asked to lie in bed and try to stay awake for as long as possible, without the aid of any gadgets, of course. Surprisingly, this group actually managed to fall asleep faster. That said, if you want to fall asleep faster, keep your eyes open and try to stay awake, without reading a book, getting on the Internet, or doing any other activity that requires physical or mental exertion. Just lie down and keep your eyes open; pretty soon, you'll find yourself drifting blissfully into sleep.

- **Keep a Pen and a Paper Beside You:** A lot of people often have bursts of insight when they're already in bed trying to sleep. By keeping a pen and a paper in your nightstand, you don't have to get up and use your computer to take down the ideas you've just harvested.

- **Brush Your Teeth After Dinner:** A lot of times, people just seem to get into the habit of eating snacks late at night, regardless of whether they're full or not. Fortunately, by brushing your teeth after dinner, late night eating becomes less appealing because of that fresh, cool breeze swirling inside your mouth.

- **Take a Hot Bath:** After taking a hot bath, your body will experience a drastic drop in core temperature, making you relaxed and drowsy.

- **Hack Your Breathing:** The 4-7-8 breathing technique is an interesting technique pioneered by Dr. Andrew Weil. This method is said to help you sleep within 60 seconds by helping oxygen fill the lungs better. You'll want to first exhale completely through your mouth, making a "whoosh" sound. Then you close your mouth and inhale through your nose while counting mentally to four. After that, hold your breath for a count of seven. After that, exhale through your mouth making the "whoosh" sound again for 8 seconds. Repeat this cycle 3 times more. Make sure that you inhale quietly through your nose and exhale loudly through your mouth.

CHAPTER 5

Sleep Disorders

With the various tips and tricks mentioned in the earlier chapters, it's easy to see how sleep can be attained with proper sleep habits and a little knowledge about the body.

But what if you're predisposed to NOT sleep well? What if your body isn't well enough to enjoy the methods described in this book? You may be fortunate enough not to have a sleeping disorder, but there are thousands of people that are struggling for a good night's sleep because their bodies simply won't let them rest.

INSOMNIA

You've probably heard this term several times with colleagues or friends that are having trouble sleeping. You might have even passed it off as them being too anxious or excited to place themselves in a state of rest.

What most people don't know about Insomnia is that is a debilitating condition that has serious repercussions on the body. It is not a phase nor is it a slight sickness that sleeping pills will cure all the time.

Definition

At the core, insomnia is a condition wherein someone has difficulty falling asleep and maintaining sleep.

You, as an adult, might have experienced this a few times in the past, especially during stressful times or before a big planned event in your life. These short, phased and finite periods of sleeplessness characterizes acute insomnia.

On the other hand, there are those who have been suffering from this condition over extended periods of time. This could be because of traumatic events or biological reasons. This is known as chronic insomnia.

Whether it's acute or chronic, one thing is always constant: your body doesn't get enough rest when you suffer from insomnia. It affects your day, mood and performance.

It was mentioned in the earlier lessons that you need quality sleep. This is represented by completing a full REM cycle in which your body paralyzes itself to prevent you from acting out in your sleep. During insomnia, people are unable to reach this stage as they have difficulty maintaining their sleep cycles or completely fail to fall asleep in general.

In today's hectic lifestyle, Insomnia has been considered as the most common sleeping disorder in the United States. More than 25 million people suffer from either acute or chronic insomnia.

Symptoms

It's difficult to tell if you have insomnia because the symptoms could easily be passed off as being tired or stressed or just the simple cause of the daily grind. With that being said, it's important to notice a pattern in these signs.

- Inability to fall asleep. Despite having the chance to lie down to get some rest, you can't seem to coerce your body into thinking that it is time to recuperate. You could either be worried about something or you feel that you still have something to do.

- Interrupted sleep. After successfully entering your first few non-REM cycles of sleep, you tend to wake up, feeling tired and irritated at the lack of rest. Even without external stimuli or disturbances, you manage to wake yourself before you arrive at your REM cycles.

- Waking up unnecessarily early. This is when you can no longer go back to sleep once you end your current cycle. You feel that you have to get started with the day despite not having enough rest.

- Errors in memorization and focus. Because of the lack of rest, you find it hard to place your mind at the right frequency needed for the work ahead of you. You also have problems remembering tasks, things and even people.

- Irritability and depression. Because of your inability to sleep well, your mood alters drastically. Since you're mostly tired by the lack of recovering sleep, you feel miserable and irritable, affecting your relationships with other people.

Besides these, there could be other symptoms connected to insomnia. You could be making a lot of mistakes at work or even worse, committing accidents while you're out and about.

The problem with undiagnosed cases of insomnia is that people tend to disregard these symptoms and just assume that they will disappear the moment that they're able to go home and get some more sleep.

This is how acute insomnia becomes chronic. Without any medical or therapeutic intervention, these symptoms just end up prolonging your suffering.

Treatment

The first step to treating insomnia is to accept that there is a pattern of sleeplessness in your daily routine. You have to stop assuming that it will all go away if you had a whole night to yourself or when the weekend sets in.

When you've recognized this pattern, don't try to solve the problem on your own. Mention it to your physician and ask for advice. Should they be knowledgeable with sleeping disorders, they may be able to make some recommendations.

This is important because you're only halfway there. Now that you know there is a problem, the next step is to finding the cause of the problem. It could be simple anxiety or something much worse. Knowing what causes insomnia allows doctors to make the right recommendations.

- Medical Problems. You might already be suffering from something else, which makes you unable to sleep. Interestingly, several other sicknesses entail insomnia as one of their symptoms. Examples of these are kidney disorders, Parkinson's disease, asthma and even cancer. You may need to go through medical examinations to find what's ailing your sleep patterns.

- Depression, anxiety and stress. These are the most common causes of insomnia, especially in chronic cases. Most people are worried about a number of things, or they could be emotionally scarred from a traumatic event from a long time. They could also be suffering from chronic stress which causes your body to feel like it is under threat despite already lying down on your bed.

- Medication. You could already be trying to solve another problem with your body by taking medicine. Your doctor will almost always ask and check your records if they've prescribed you anything that will cause you to lose sleep. It's also a good idea to take a look at your vitamins and supplements and ask about them. In other rare cases, even birth control pills have been found to cause insomnia in some women.

- Other sleep problems. At the core, insomnia could be a symptom or a disorder in itself. Sometimes, it also means you have other sleeping problems that require additional attention. You could be suffering from sleep apnea or jet-lag or even a deviation from your circadian rhythm.

Once you zero in on the cause, it's a matter of applying various methods to coax your body into relaxing. Just like the causes of insomnia, treatments can also vary.

Acupuncture for Insomnia

Surprisingly, there is now direct scientific evidence linking acupuncture to sleep problems. Studies done in 2004 have shown that acupuncture has directly caused better nights for people who suffered from insomnia.

Based on the studies, a control group that was subjected to individual sessions of acupuncture were shown to have more levels of melatonin during sleep. This, in turn, led to longer periods of undisturbed sleep. You will know melatonin as a hormone that is closely related to your sleeping and waking cycles. When it is present in the system, it prepares the body for a period of resting and recuperation.

But you can't just start sticking needles into yourself. This is an old art but it is one that requires an expert. Fortunately, there are many services that have online portals that allow you to book a session or give you access to their facilities and staff.

In case you're still in the dark about this, acupuncture is the therapeutic process of sticking long, thin needles in various parts of the body. This may sound painful and unusual at first, but these sessions have been claimed to be pain-free.

Based on ancient Chinese medical beliefs, acupuncture was initially meant to cure disease by targeting specific acupressure points in the body with needles. This, in turn, would release internal energy in the body and allow good energy to flow in through the right channels.

This system has changed over the years but is still being practiced by many experts in the field.

It is important to remember that acupuncture still remains as a complementary method to tried and proven methods. This isn't a cure in itself, and should always be taken under the supervision of a doctor.

JET LAG

What is just considered as a side-effect of flying through different time zones could be something that drastically affects the quality of your sleep.

Jet lag is a condition wherein you cannot sleep well and experience other discomforts when you pass through several time zones. Frequent flyers talk about this condition when they make several breaks through different continents, each with their own time zones.

People who suffer from jet lag usually find it hard to sleep or become really sleepy at inappropriate times of the country in which they've arrived. Because of the different time zones, you could still be greeted by the morning sun after a twelve-hour flight that took off in the early morning.

When your body expects it to be night time with the absence of sunlight but is greeted hours later by the same sunlight despite a long amount of time passing, then it's bound to cause an imbalance within your natural rhythm. This could lead to the following things:

- Irritability

- Fatigue

- Loss of Focus

- Lethargy

- Headaches

- Digestive problems

- Insomnia

Should you experience these symptoms after a long flight, that means your body is reeling from the effects of the changing zones. This means you need to get quality sleep in order to reset your functions.

Treatment

For most cases, jet lag serves as a temporary drawback to the wonders of travel. Give yourself a day of rest and your body will have completely adjusted to the new time zone.

With that being said, there are a few more remedies available to help you better adapt to this phenomenon:

- If you're staying in a new country for several days, give yourself a few days of rest, equal to the number of time zones you'll be crossing. If you're only staying abroad for a short while, try to maintain your original sleep schedule and put up with the initial discomforts of your destination. It's better than adjusting once more when you come back home.

- Adapt to your Destination. If your destination is several hours ahead, train yourself to sleep the same time the people there sleep, even if you're not yet there. Use an international clock to keep track of the time differences as you adjust your sleeping patterns. You won't be shocked by jet lag as much if you've been changing your sleep schedule before your plan leaves.

- Avoid in-flight alcohol and caffeine. These substances will only either give you a rush or a down, which are both unnecessary as you pass through different time zones. These will only tarnish the quality of sleep you get while you're in-flight.

- Use Melatonin. Think of this as one of the few cases where a sleeping aid is necessary. As you approach the time zone of your destination, you need to coincide your sleep pattern with theirs. This may be difficult especially when you're going through a large time difference. Melatonin will help ease your body to sleep during irregular hours as you try to match the time zone of your destination.

- Keep yourself very hydrated. Because of the shifting nature of your biological clock, you can never tell when your body will be in a resting or active state. Whatever state that may be, you need to be sure there is plenty of water in your system. Since jet lag may cause a change in your bowel movement as well, it pays to stay well-hydrated during long trips so that you land with an intact stomach and a healthy glow.

- Use the Sun. Don't just keep those window shutters closed. You will want to get sunlight even while you're flying, especially when you're approaching your destination. If you're arriving at night, it's best to keep the shutters closed.

These methods have been used by many professionals in the aviation industry to keep themselves healthy despite their frequent passing through different time zones.

RESTLESS LEG SYNDROME

Also known as RLS, this condition strangely finds its way as a disorder that affects your sleep.

You may be wondering how something that affects your lower appendage meddles with a good night's sleep. At the very core, RLS affects the nervous system. It creates uncomfortable sensations in the leg. These sensations vary from the feeling of something crawling up your legs, pain, pins, limpness and even itchiness.

These sensations happen even if there's nothing actually happening in your legs. They're all in the mind. Imagine these sensations happening to you as you sleep. That is how RLS affects the quality and length of your rest. People that suffer from RLS wake up in the middle of night to move and scratch their legs even if there's nothing wrong with them.

Causes

Interestingly, RLS also serves as a symptom of other disorders and diseases. People that suffer from Parkinson's and Diabetes have been known to show symptoms of RLS. Kidney sicknesses and deficiencies with iron have also been known to share space with RLS.

Some antidepressants have also been known to induce RLS, especially when taken regularly. When taken despite showing symptoms of RLS, these drugs may end up worsening the symptoms; making pain more intense and what not.

Treatment

Since RLS is connected to other diseases, treating those conditions directly contribute to easing the symptoms of RLS. This takes coordination with your physician based on what's wrong with you.

If your medication is causing your discomfort, you need to check your prescriptions and ask your specialist for alternatives that don't bring the same side-effect.

There are also cases wherein RLS sets in after you stop taking a certain medication. This is your body getting used to a now-normal routine without the assistance of your medicine.

On another note, pampering your legs a little doesn't hurt your chances of avoiding RLS when you sleep. The following tips may be done at home to help with the symptoms:

- Getting a massage. Take note that RLS is a condition of the nervous system. Your brain sends signals to your legs to feel a certain way despite the absence of any stimuli. Feeding your nerves a relaxing massage is one way of curbing the tendency of feeling pain. It's hard to trick your legs into feeling pain when they're relaxed and pampered.

- Hot and Cold Packs. This choice depends on your plans for the next day. If you're aiming for a cool night's rest, a cold pack for the legs is a great way to lower your temperature for the night. If you're already suffering from leg pains before going to bed, a hot pack will help blood circulation to bring more oxygen to your lower regions.

- Relaxis. This is known as a vibrating pad. One very unique thing about RLS is that is affects the nerves of the legs without damaging the external portion of your appendage. One way to interrupt these attacks is to provide an external stimulus to the legs. Give them something to experience to overload the nerves in the legs. That's what a vibrating pad does. Your brain won't have the time to send the wrong signals to the legs if your legs are already experiencing light vibrations as you sleep.

Unfortunately, there is no one proven cure to completely get rid of RLS. The best thing that you can do is to ensure your sleep is undisturbed by the "phantom pains" brought about by such a condition.

NARCOLEPSY

If there are disorders that cause you to avoid and disrupt sleep, there are also orders that make you sleepy when you're not supposed to be. One such example is narcolepsy.

Characterized by being excessively sleepy during the day, narcolepsy plagues 1 out of 2000 people in the United States. It may sound like a rare disorder but it's one that doesn't just affects your day. It affects your nights as well.

People who suffer narcolepsy are almost devoid of active function. Despite having the right amount of sleep, they still become very lethargic during the waking hours of the day. They tend to fall asleep easily in the afternoon, despite there being no chance to sleep well. They may even fall asleep right in the middle of certain activities.

For patients with narcolepsy, their bodies can't really distinguish when it's time to be awake or resting. That line has been blurred. This is why they exhibit symptoms of sleepiness when they're supposed to be out and about.

On top of these problems when they wake, their bodies can't really recognize when it's time to rest. This causes them to wake up in the middle of night, supposedly to do something. These disruptions in their sleep and awake cycles centers on an anomaly inside your hypothalamus.

Causes

The main culprit behind narcolepsy is the absence of a certain chemical produced by the brain known as hypocretin. Think of this as the "wake up" substance in the body.

When the hypothalamus creates hypocretin, the body is lead to believe that the time for resting is over and it is time to increase brain activity, metabolic rate as well as heart rate. These things are what keeps us up in the morning after we get a good night's sleep.

For a person with narcolepsy, either their hypothalamus is damaged or is not functioning properly, causing it to fail to produce this important chemical. Without this chemical, the body has no way to knowing when it's time to kick it into high gear or to just keep things mellow and sleepy.

Treatment

Sadly, narcolepsy is similar to RLS in the sense that there hasn't been a proven cure to fully rid someone of the disorder. The delicate nature of the hypothalamus makes it hard to cure.

Despite that, there are some methods to alleviate the symptoms and to provide better energy throughout the day.

- Forcefully boost your metabolism. If your body is incapable of distinguishing awake and sleep time, you can jump start things on your own by drinking plenty of water during the day. This will force your body to kick up its processing speeds to meet the demands of your day. About 16 ounces will do the trick

- Engage in cardio workouts. What better way to tell the body that it's time to be up and about than by giving your heart a literal run for its money? Engaging in exercise that elevates heart rate is a great way to keep yourself alive and awake and enthusiastic during crucial parts of your work day.

- Avoid processed foods. Since your body has a sleeping metabolic rate, ingesting food that takes time to digest is only going to make things hard for you. You'll end up with clogged arteries and other disorders to complement your narcolepsy.

- Change your multivitamins. The good thing about vitamins is that you can change them depending on your need. You don't just need a simple boost of vitamin C everday. Sometimes, you need iron as well. Speak to your doctor about vitamins that boost your energy and keep you up when it is most needed.

- STILL stay away from caffeine. Just because you're sleepy when you're not supposed to, that doesn't mean coffee is going to work wonders for your waking hours. It still won't help. After you burn out the caffeine in your system, your body will revert to narcoleptic symptoms at a later time.

- Use the Sun. Take advantage of your body's sensitivity to sunlight. During the morning, take a quick stroll in the morning sun to give your body a wake-up call.

Take note that these steps should be taken along with a trip to your doctor. They will be prescribing you with alternative medicines to help you deal with these symptoms. They may not eliminate your narcolepsy, but they'll make your day-to-day easier to manage.

DELAYED SLEEP PHASE DISORDER

Most commonly found in teens, this disorder stems from an abnormality with your circadian rhythm. Your body's natural metabolic rate and energy levels peak and drop at inappropriate times.

For people that suffer from this, they find it impossible to sleep in the wee hours of the morning. This is much different from a "night person" that just likes staying up late. These are people that cannot go to sleep because their bodies won't let them.

This is more of a problem with the circadian cycle of a person. It is not in synch with the body, causing a great delay in the things that are supposed to happen. People who suffer from this feel sleepy and ready for bed in the morning because of these delays. When everyone needs to go to bed, they feel like their day is just about to start.

Causes

This problem could be caused by an unhealthy development of bad sleep hygiene. Getting used to unusual hours of waking and sleeping could cause your body to adjust accordingly, changing its whole circadian clock to accommodate your unusual sleeping behavior. When this adjustment has been solidified, it becomes even harder to overcome.

This is why this disorder is seen in mostly teenagers because of their natural tendencies to stay up late. Despite that, it can also happen to adults given the proper conditions. When this happens, a solidified circadian clock with wrong bearings becomes difficult to change without drastic lifestyle changes.

Treatment

One of the best methods for restoring the circadian rhythm to normal is the use of natural light. This is also known as Bright Light Therapy.

As the name implies, the method uses artificial light to coax the body into making changes it its circadian clock in order to follow a normal routine. It's also called phototherapy. Here, patients go about critical portions of the day with a device called a light box. This box emits a bright light that emulates the brightness of natural light from the outside.

With the help of a specialist, you will be subjected to this box at certain times of the day; ideally, you want these times to be regular waking hours. Since the body follow a different cycle from the norm, the light emitted by the box will serve as a strong reminder to the body to stay active.

During sleeping hours when it is time to rest, the light box is not used. When done consistently, your body will start to build a dependence on the light from the box, changing peaks and dips in your alertness levels. During times without the box, the body will get ready for sleep.

By sticking with the therapy, you can "reset" your circadian clock and restore your sleeping habits to normal.

Fortunately, bright light therapy is also used to remedy many other types of circadian clock disorders.

CHAPTER 6

Stress and Sleeptress

In today's very hectic life and fast-paced demands, it's easy to lose sleep due to stress advice by changing some of your sleeping habits..

The problem here is, how much do you know about stress? Are you really experiencing stress or just a bad day? Are you aware of how stress affects your sleeping patterns?

STRESS DEFINED

As an adult, you've probably had a big share of low days wherein the demands seem like too much. When your brain recognizes the fact that your job, livelihood or health is in danger, it goes into your stress response.

At the very core, stress triggers your body into a state wherein it perceives a threat. Since your body cannot discern the kind of threat, it prepares you to either flee from the threat or to engage the threat (in combat).

In that state, your brain tells the body to create adrenaline and to increase blood pressure. This allows more oxygen to get to your muscles in preparation to deal with the threat. That's good if you were about to run from an assailant or a wild animal.

But what if the threat was a big report that was due in the next 24 hours at work? That's not something a boost of adrenaline will fix. What if it was a client meeting with a notorious prospect that's been known to be harsh on people? Heightened senses don't work well with that.

Remember that your body is not able to recognize the nature of your threat. All it knows is that it is under attack because of your state of mind. This is where modern day stress comes in. Imagine being in such a defensive state all day; with adrenaline in your systems and decreased brain activity because of a lack of oxygen.

Imagine yourself trying to go to bed in that state. Wouldn't it be impossible to relax when your body thinks that it is under threat? That is what stress does to the body in relation to your sleeping patterns.

STRESS IN YOUR LIFE

You may have felt like that at least a few times in your life; when there was a big demand that was looming inside your head for a whole night. It's very difficult to get sleep no matter how relaxing and conducive the environment may be.

What makes things worse is that this prolonged state of defense takes its toll on the body. On top of trouble sleeping, you could end up with other health complications.

Are you constantly worrying about something that is about to happen? Is there something bothering your state of mind to the point that you even worry about it when you're about to sleep? If the answer is yes, then you might need a different approach instead of trying various sleep hacks.

STRESS BUSTING FOR SLEEP

The first thing you need to know about stress is that it is a physiological state of emergency. The main goal to busting stress is to give your body the impression that you are, in fact, not in danger. When the sense of danger has dissipated, so will your stress signals.

Meditation

Since your problem is your state of mind, altering your thoughts through meditation is one of the best ways to win back stress-deprived sleep.

The best thing about meditation is that it is a personal experience, which means that there is no one proper way to do it. With the many methods available right now, it's just a matter of finding something that works for you. If it allows you to relax and gain control of the situation, then that's what will work for you.

One of the most popular methods of meditation is mindfulness meditation. This is the complete shift of focus from your personal thoughts to the immediate environment. This form of meditation can be done anywhere and in almost any position. Plus, it's a great way to change your perspective from what's bothering you to something completely neutral. In the process, you allow your body to relax and return to a normal state, ready for rest.

Aromatherapy

This isn't just a trend among homeowners that want their houses to smell nice for visitors. It's a clinically-proven method of using various fragrances to trigger certain portions of the brain to release certain hormones that help the body shift from a state of danger to a state of calmness.

As studies have shown, certain smells from different herbs and flowers are known to create certain feelings in people, allowing them to calm down in otherwise hectic environments.

Fortunately, aromatherapy can be done with some of the simplest methods. All you need are essential oils of the fragrances you want to use. Some of the best examples for calming oils are lavender and chamomile as well as ylang-ylang.

You can either use a diffuser or simply apply the oil to your palms and neck to start calming down. The essential oils take care of the rest. Another good thing about these oils is that there are hundreds upon hundreds of available oils to choose from. You may be surprised at what you may find at your nearest fragrance store.

Communication

You may not have seen a connection, but talking about your stressors and stress responses is one of the best ways to deal with stress. The great thing about communication is that it serves as a catalyst for changing your perspective on things. There's something about relaying your problems that allows you to see your concerns in a more objective manner.

You may or may not get advice about your stress when you talk to your friends or family about your problems. What's important is that you are able to speak your mind and get some form of relief from your troubles.

Communication also doesn't have to happen right before you go to bed. It can be done at work or when you have the time. Once you've taken a load off your chest, the chances of you being able to relax increase by the time you're ready for bed.

CHAPTER 7

Understanding Your Circadian Rhythm

Having a firm understanding of your circadian cycle is important. It's sometimes called your circadian rhythm or circadian cycle. Whatever name you use, it refers to the same thing.

Think of this cycle as your "supposed" natural daily cycle. Humans should be doing certain things at certain parts of the day. This is not because it's the right thing to do, but because our bodies are better-tuned to do certain things at certain times.

The Circadian Cycle Explained

This cycle doesn't just pertain to your sleeping habits. Everything from resting to eating is also a part of this cycle.

This is because your body also follows a rhythm depending on the time of day. Have you ever experienced scenes of drowsiness at certain stages of the day? That's probably your biological clock playing along with your circadian cycle.

You have dips and peaks of energy due to this rhythm. All of this happens because of your hypothalamus. This is a very important region in your nervous system that coordinates your organs and your enzymes.

At certain parts of the day, your hypothalamus sends various signals to your body to either increase the need for sleep or activity. These needs depend on what your body perceives as the time of day; and no, your actual house clock has nothing to do with that.

Your hypothalamus takes cues from how long you've been awake and how much sunlight you're getting. Have you ever noticed why you get better sleep when you sleep at night instead of during the day? This is because the hypothalamus prepares the body to sleep when there is no light. That's how it knows that it's time to rest.

Circadian Sleep Pattern Disruptors

One reason why you're having trouble sleeping is because you're probably not synchronized with your natural circadian rhythm. Back-track to the past weeks and try to see if you've established a bad pattern of sleeping habits.

Have you gone to sleep and woken up at the same time everyday? Including the weekends? Take note that this is rhythm. It has to be consistent.

There are some people who also don't have control over their sleeping patterns. People who work graveyard shifts or those who fly often that experience jetlag sometimes have a hard time following their natural sleep patterns.

There are also certain prescription drugs used for lifetime medication that can cause a disruption in natural sleeping patterns. Depending on your current medical condition, something you're already taking could already be disrupting your cycle.

Take note that your circadian rhythm is sensitive to the presence of light, whether it be organic or synthetic. That means the presence of too much light at night could also be affecting your ability to sleep well. Do you work late into the night with a lot of light?

Following the Rhythm

In line with getting things back on track, restoring your sleep cycle requires a few new habits that will reinforce your body's adherence to its natural cycle.

It was mentioned in the earlier chapters that maintaining a normal and consistent sleep pattern is the first step. Going to bed when night comes and waking up when the sun comes up is the backbone of your natural cycle. Following that, there are other complementary methods to coax your body into inducing sleep easily.

- Soak in the sun. When morning comes, don't just immediately hit the showers and head on to work. Take a few minutes to soak in the early morning sun. Besides the good vitamin D boost, you're also giving your body an energy boost by alerting your hypothalamus that there's plenty of light and it's time to work. This will give you the energy you need for the day and will give your body a good excuse to power down when you get home once the day ends.

- Lights out at night. If basking in the sun is good during the early morning, then going all black-out during the night works the same way. Pick a safe time to hit the sheets and make sure that there is no light in your room. If it's still bright outside because of your neighbors, install some thick curtains to block out everything.

- Sleep like a weekday everyday. This means maintaining the same sleeping pattern even on the weekends. If you can go through a whole week with the same sleeping patterns, you won't have any trouble finding sleep any day of the week moving forward.

- Heavy meals for breakfast and light meals for the evening. It's not just your sleeping patterns that have to change. Your eating patterns should also coincide with your cycle. Your body digests better in the morning. That should give you plenty of energy for the day. At night, stick to a small meal before capping off the day. This will help you avoid digestive interruptions in the middle of the night. Your body's digestive operations aren't as hot as they are in the morning because your body is getting prepared for a long period of rest.

- Avoid the spicy and the caffeinated. You may love these food items but you want to lay off them in the evening. These are disruptors to your natural rhythm because they give your hypothalamus the impression that you're about to start your day.

- Adjust your other daily activities. Do you jog in the evening? That may be tricking your brain into thinking that it's still morning and you still need to be up and about. Move these activities to the morning when your energy and metabolism are at their peak.

If Things Go Wrong

You have learned about Delayed Sleep Phase Disorder in an earlier chapter of this book. That is an example of a disrupted circadian cycle. Take note that this is not the only way that you can damage your internal clock and completely mess up your sleeping patterns.

Did you know that you could also end up going to bed earlier than most people? Even with the sun still out? That's known as Advanced Sleep Phase Disorder. It also stems from an irregularity in your circadian cycle.

When you start keeping unhygienic sleeping habits, your body will start adjusting to these changes in anticipation of a new sleeping pattern. This is why it's vital for you to maintain good sleeping habits to keep your circadian clock in check.

CHAPTER 8

Sleep Cheats

By this time I already remembered the golden rule of sleep: you need to get the right kind at the right quantity at the right time for it to matter.

But what if that's not an option? With the demands of modern-day jobs and families, it's sometimes impossible to squeeze in 8-9 hours of sleep in preparation for the next day. Worse, these instances happen when there is something big the following day.

What if it was your job to wake up and forsaken hours in the morning because you're on-call? What if the entirety of your work day takes place in the graveyard shift? Various external causes could contribute to you losing sleep by no fault of yours; but that doesn't mean you have to put up with the lethargy and low energy.

POLYPHASIC SLEEP

Also known as Uberman's Sleep Schedule, this method of sleeping changes your sleeping patterns but doesn't cut out on the necessary quality rest that your body needs.

The usual pattern of sleeping is known as biphasic. That means there are two phases for sleep within a 24-hour block. With that being said, polyphasic sleep pertains to sleeping several times a day.

Polyphasic Sleep Vs. Napping

This is completely different from napping in the middle of the day. The goal of polyphasic sleep is to trick your brain into noticing a new pattern in your sleep pattern that it forces itself to work faster in a shorter time span.

Take note that naps are only supposed to take no more than 20 minutes. Anything after that and your body will start diving into a full sleep cycle. With polyphasic sleep, you want your body to make that dive but only for about 2 hours.

The core approach of polyphasic sleeping is to break down your full resting period for a day into 4 to 6 sleep periods, each being about 2 hours long. This may sound like a crude approach to cutting corners on sleep, but it's a crude method that works.

How it Works

Take note that the body doesn't necessarily have to experience a full 8 hours of sleep to start recuperating and healing. It just has to be in the right state while you sleep. Normally, that takes time as you go through each cycle.

With polyphasic sleep, you start telling your body that you will no longer be able to get a full 8 hours of sleep. Instead, you're replacing your full 8 hours with smaller 2-hour chunks that happen frequently throughout the day.

Depending on how long your body takes to get the hint, you could be looking at 2 weeks until your body realizes that a full 8 hour block of sleeping is never happening.

When this happens, your body will begin to adjust to your new pattern of sleeping by injecting as much brain activity in your new (and limited) sleep time as possible. This will allow you to wake up refreshed and energized after a mere two hours of sleep.

Benefits

Naturally, this method works great for people who have very little control over the time they get to sleep. Professionals that need to be on-call for emergencies will now have the energy to do what they have to do without sacrificing their good night's sleep.

This sleeping pattern also allows you to do more within the day, especially if you're more inclined to do things when you're supposed to be sleeping. The flexibility that this method provides you allows you more space in which to plot out your daily activities instead of squeezing everything into a single day.

Disadvantages

Primarily, getting used to the new sleeping pattern will not be easy. From a regular biphasic sleep pattern, you're going to force yourself to divide that into smaller chunks. That will mean sleeping in inappropriate times of the day as well as making yourself wake up in the middle of the night.

These things will initially drain you and make you very cranky and uncooperative. As good as the method sounds, it doesn't come without its share of drawbacks.

If you're on a regular work shift and you value your daytime over your nights, polyphasic sleeping may not be the best option for you. Take a good look at your circumstances before trying this one out.

CAFFEINE-ASSISTED NAPPING

It has been mentioned in the earlier chapters that you should stay away from caffeinated drinks before going to bed. This is because it doesn't help your body relax when it's supposed to be powering down.

Interestingly, caffeine may be able to help you nap instead of helping you go to sleep at night. This is because caffeine takes about 20 minutes before it is absorbed into the bloodstream.

Coincide your caffeine consumption with a nap and you end up with a built-in wake-up mechanism! If you take a cup of coffee right before your slide off into your afternoon nap, you'll give the caffeine just enough time to work while giving you a mini-boost in energy and focus.

You just want to be careful about becoming dependent on caffeine when it comes to waking up. On top of depending on coffee in the morning, you will have another reason to look for coffee in the afternoon or whenever you need to take a nap.

PROGRESSIVE MUSCLE RELAXATION

Another trick that you can do is a form of stretching right before going to bed. Progressive muscle relaxation is a method of causing the muscles to ease out no matter how hectic the day was for you.

Interestingly, it merely consists of a two-step process and can be done on almost any part of the body. This chapter will teach you a full body approach to ensure that you're wholly relaxed before hitting the sheets.

Start by finding some alone time. This makes pre-bedtime one of the best opportunities. You don't necessarily have to be lying down but it's much better than sitting.

Once you've found a nice spot, quiet your thoughts and focus on relaxing. Your muscle relaxation session can begin anywhere you want. You can start from head to toe or vice versa. Here, you will start with the neck.

Phase 1: Applying Tension

Before there can be relaxation, there has to be something from which to feel relief. The first part of muscle relaxation is applying tension to the muscles. Fortunately, you don't have to lift anything. Simply bending or contracting your muscles serves as a good form of tension.

With the neck, bend your head to one side, keeping it there until you feel a strain develop in the area. That is how you apply tension within that area.

Phase 2: Relaxation

Once you start to feel a strain, release yourself from that position and return to a more comfortable posture. At this point, feel your muscles relax as you go back to your original position. That's the basis of Progressive muscle relaxation.

The back and forth between tension and relaxation will allow you to shift your thoughts from sleeping to the comfort brought about by the second phase.

Of course, you're still just talking about the neck area. Once you're done with the neck, move to the other parts of your body; being the shoulders, arms, hands so on and so forth.

Clench your fists as hard as you can or twist your torso until you feel a strain develop in the area. That's the signal to release and relax the muscles. Think of it as a warm up before sleeping.

In this state, the relaxation of your muscles will make it easier for you to fall asleep because of the feeling of comfort brought about by the stretching and tensing.

CHAPTER 9

Snoring

Almost heard every time someone talks about sleeping, snoring has had its share of jokes and gags that may make you think it's not a big deal. What may be just an annoying habit could be a sign that there's something wrong with your sleep habits and it may just be the start of something worse.

What is a Snore?

People have described snores as someone breaking boards with their mouths as they sleep. Others have said it sounds like a dying pig being murdered in the wee hours of the morning. No matter how it sounds, a snore is a vibration somewhere in your throat.

Simply put, snoring happens when a blockade in your mouth and nasal passageways vibrates as you breathe. It could be swollen tissue, fat or even some foreign object that found its way into your air passages.

This is a condition anyone could have, regardless of age and gender; but is mostly seen in older men. Depending on what's obstructing the flow of air in your mouth and nose, snoring could disrupt your sleep via the following ways.

- Your snoring could wake you up in the middle of your rest. Because you have a blockade in the air paths, it's very likely that a change in position might cause you to choke in your sleep. Of course, the lack of breathe will wake you, but will require you to start your whole sleep cycle from the beginning.

- Even if you're still able to breathe, the blockade still diminishes the amount of oxygen you take in per breath. Your body makes do with what is available and may not give you quality rest. Thus, there's a large chance you wake up tired and in need of more sleep.

- Finally, severe cases of snoring could eventually lead to sleep apnea, which is even worse. You could end up forcing yourself to sleep light even when you need deep sleep because you're afraid of gasping for air in the middle of the night.

These factors are some of the reasons that snoring gets its own chapter in this book. It's a much-overlooked aspect of sleep that most people pass off as an irritating habit that "they just have to live with".

Causes of Snoring

Depending on the nature of what blocks the air passages in your mouth and nose, several things could be contributing to your snoring condition. Here are some common culprits.

- Allergy Attacks. You may be sleeping in a dusty room or ate something you shouldn't have before going to bed. Your allergic reaction could cause a swelling in the throat, sinuses or nostrils which could be the blockades to your oxygen intake.

- Obesity. Your body doesn't just store fat in your gust and your thighs. It can sometimes cause other parts of your body to fatten out of proportion; like your throat tissues. Some cases of obesity have been known to give people enlarged throat tissues and even tonsils. These could end up blocking the air you breathe.

- Weak Muscles. Especially in the throat area. You may not be obese or suffering from allergic attacks, but your throat muscles may be too weak and relaxed. When this happens, there is a large chance of them sinking back into the back of your throat, blocking the air as you breathe in your sleep.

- Genetic Reasons. You could have just been born with a long uvula or soft palate. These are parts of your mouth that usually lie at the back of the neck, right before the throat. When these tissues are too large for their own good, there's a good tendency for them to vibrate against each other when you breathe.

Whether it's your natural state or an allergy attack, the important thing to realize is that snoring is a medical condition. That means there are ways to remedy this condition. It should not be dismissed as a pet peeve, rather a sign that there is something wrong that needs correction.

HOW TO CURE SNORING

In order to curb your snoring, it's important to determine what's causing you to make those awful sounds when you sleep. It could be one of those three reasons mentioned earlier. Consulting a physician is a great idea to zero in on the cause.

Once you've found out the cause, you can try a few remedies to see if they can help alleviate the problem.

- Get a humidifier. If the cause of your snoring is an allergic reaction, you have to sanitize the air in your bedroom. There could be free particles that are finding their way into your nostrils which could cause them to swell with irritation. A humidifier will help clean the air that you breathe and allow you to avoid inhaling anything that could trigger your reactions.

- Sleeping on your sides. If the cause of your snoring has something to do with the size of your tongue and the other tissues at the back of the mouth, changing positions while sleeping could do the trick. As opposed to lying on your back, lying on your side doesn't allow the back of your tongue to recede back into the throat where it can obstruct your breathing. Instead, you're causing it to fall to the sides.

- Go up. At least in terms of your head. Ensuring your head is at least four inches above the body makes gravity work in your favor. This works the same way as sleeping on your sides. You ensure that the tissues in the mouth and the throat don't relax into your air passages.

- Clean your nose with saline. This will help clear your nostrils of irritants before you turn off the lights; provided that it's your allergies that are causing you to snore. It's a good complement to your nightly bath before sleeping if you're practicing the other tips mentioned in this book.

- Stay away from sedatives. Or anything else that artificially induces relaxation unless advised by your doctor. The thing with sedatives and sleeping pills is that they don't just cause your mind to relax, they cause the whole body to relax. That includes the muscles in your throat which could end up blocking the oxygen you inhale.

- Use snoring mouthpieces. These are effective if the cause of your snoring is the shape and size of your mouth, jaw, tongue and other tissues. These mouthpieces were designed to position your mouth in such a way that the back of your tongue doesn't slide into the back of your throat. You don't have to change positions or sleep on your side for them to work.

Take note that these are just home remedies that you can try on your own. If in the case that nothing seems to stop the snoring, it's time to approach a doctor for more options. From there, you could be looking at clinical and even surgical approaches to get rid of the problem once and for all.

From using lasers to trim tissues and radio waves to collapse walls of fat, the doctors will be able to make the best choice for you. The goal of surgical treatments is to permanently remove the obstruction from your mouth and nose without hampering their normal functions.

CHAPTER 10

Sleep and Dreams

Discussions always present in conversations about sleep. Considered as one of the strangest doorways to the human psyche, dreams have developed an aura mysticism and spirituality that seems to have bridged the gap between psychology and the future.

What are Dreams?

Answers could vary from person to person, depending on who you ask. Some will say that dreams are visions that your memories generate at the peak of brain activity. Some people will say that they are reflections of your subconscious thoughts which were given freedom during sleep.

Scientifically, dreams are pictures, thoughts, feelings and stimuli that people experience as they sleep. They could be events that play themselves out as someone sleeps. They usually occur during REM cycles where brain activity is heightened. Because we are unconscious when we sleep, dreaming is deemed as an involuntary action. We cannot control or dictate when we dream or not.

The contents (or events) that take place in a dream are also involuntary instances. When we dream, we cannot dictate what we dream about.

This doesn't stop us from dreaming anything from the range of mundane to the unbelievable.

Much discussion has been channeled towards interpreting dreams and giving them meaning. Many psychologists and spiritualists draw a connection between dreaming and what we want for ourselves.

Connection to Sleep

There isn't any evidence to point out that dreaming means you are getting good quality sleep. Although experts have pointed out that dreaming is enhanced brain activity at the right time during sleep, not everyone that dreams ends up feeling well rested in the morning.

With that much being said about the benefits of dreaming, the connection between dreaming and sleeping may take a turn if you're not having good dreams. These are known as nightmares.

Nightmares

It was said that we could dream about anything because this is an involuntary action on our end as we go through our sleep cycles. This means we could dream of something very boring, very nice, and even something terrible.

Nightmares are dreams about disturbing things that completely ruin our sleep cycles because they wake us up in the middle of the night. These could be embarrassing moments, scary movies we've seen during the day or even traumatic experiences that are being relived in the mind.

Whatever the content may be, they are a real threat to you getting a good night's sleep; especially if you have an active imagination and if you dream often. It even affects you for the rest of the day if you're the kind of person that can easily recall what they dream about. Unfortunately, unpleasant dreams are the easiest to remember because they jolt us awake right in the middle of our sleep cycles.

What's even worse is that nightmares may even prevent us from going back to sleep because we end up being flustered or disturbed by what we dreamt of.

Studies have shown that children are more prone to experiencing nightmares. This might be attributed to their tendency to be easily influenced by what happens around them.

It is also possible for adults to have nightmares as well. Depending on the kind of nightmare being experienced, a full adult could be known to suffer anxiety, depression and other psychological problems because of the recurrence of nightmares.

What Causes Nightmares?

Some experts theorize that nightmares were built in as a defense mechanism that prepares us to tackle deep issues that require out attention.

Although that hypothesis hasn't been proven yet, experts can safely point out that stress and anxiety are some of the natural culprits behind nightmares. Usually, people who are constantly worried about things tend to bring their worries with them as they sleep.

Another cause for nightmares is in terms of content. People that have gone through traumatic experiences are usually revisited by their experiences when they sleep. From losing a loved one to being involved in a major accident, people that have experienced terrifying incidents in real life are more likely to relive them in their dreams.

On a simpler note, increasing your brain activity right before going to be also increases the chance of unpleasant dreams. Taking in coffee, smoking and even drinking alcohol before going to bed are all considered as catalysts for unpleasant nights in dreamland.

How to prevent Nightmares

Truth be told, dreams are much of an unexplored and poorly-researched area. Dreams mean different things for people and experts. There are healthy people that suffer from nightmares. There are sickly people that dream peacefully at night. There are also people that complain about never dreaming at all despite their health conditions.

To prevent nightmares, experts point to the direction of stress relief. If you're suffering from regular nightmares, there's a large chance that there's something bothering you during your waking hours.

- You could be suffering from chronic stress as well. Revert back to the chapter on stress for effective tips on clearing your mind. With a clear mind with nothing to worry about, the chances of your brain destabilizing neuron connections with those memories and emotions are highly unlikely.

- You should also take a look at the medications that you have. There are drugs that tamper with your brain and its capacity to make neuron connections while you sleep. Talk to your doctor about their recommendations.

- If your nightmares stem from a traumatic experience, take note of how long you've been suffering from them. You may need some professional help to get you to accept these things. Talking to your family and friends will also help with the moving on process. Good sleep helps you move on from traumatic events better. Restoring your sleep is one good way to ease your suffering and help you accept things.

- Avoid snacking late at night. It may not sound connected to your dreams but eating when you should be sleeping forces your metabolic rate to go up. When this happens, brain activity also increases. This could lead to dreams which could end up in nightmares.

- Start a dream journal. It's a very therapeutic process. Take note that dreams are hard to remember when you try to recall them in the middle of the day. Writing about your dreams should take place the moment you wake up, when memories of that dream are raw and still haven't left your waking mind. With a dream journal, you'll be able to zero in on what part of your dreams is upsetting, helping you deal with it in real life.

Conclusion

Thank you again for purchasing this book!

I hope this book was able to help you to understand the basics of sleep, what happens in your body when you sleep, and how to get restorative, uninterrupted sleep every night.

As you sleep your way to good health, you should notice a couple of simple, subtle, but powerful changes starting to happen in your daily life:

- You can get away with less sleep – People with busy lifestyles often compromise their sleeping schedules and try to get away with as little as 5 hours of sleep every night. This causes them to work less efficiently and eventually crash out of fatigue. Surprisingly, though, with the right context, habits, and bio-hacks, it's possible for you to get away with 5-6 hours of sleep once in a while without causing you to be groggy the entire day. Studies also show that certain people are genetically programmed to require less sleep cycles, so if you're one of those people fortunate enough to require only 5-6 hours of sleep, the tips and tricks provided in this book will help you make sure that the small amount of sleep you need provides you with enough energy to face the day.

- Your injuries heal faster – Deep sleep is where healing happens at an accelerated rate. As you get better sleep every night, you'll notice that injuries actually get better a lot faster.

- You may not need coffee anymore! – A lot of people go for coffee because they have a hard time pulling themselves out of bed each morning. However, remember that, in the past, our ancestors didn't need coffee to run a couple of miles every day, our bodies are wired to be energized in the morning and sleepy at night. People often drink coffee when they get inadequate sleep but still need to perform complex thinking tasks in the morning, but by following the tips and tricks in this book, your body will be able to self-caffeinate in the morning, and although the energy you get may not feel like the unnatural jittery buzz you get from coffee, it'll be stable, and it'll be with you the whole day. The best part is, your body won't develop tolerance to natural energy!

To effectively use the tips and tricks this book provides, you'll have to understand first that oftentimes, the reason it's so difficult to break the bad habits that have seeped into your day-to-day activities isn't because you're too weak, but because your brain's energy is zapped and you're running on autopilot. Remember that all habits can be reprogrammed if attacked in the correct and consistent manner.

Although the information provided in this book is up-to-date when it was gathered, discoveries are made in the medical field every day. If you find yourself not getting a good night's sleep despite following the tips and tricks provided in this book, you may need to tweak and modify these guidelines and augment them with information you may stumble upon in the future. You'll also want to consult your physician, especially with the supplements this book lists, and especially if you're currently taking form of medication, as certain supplements may prevent some medications from working properly.

Now that you know the most effective ways to sleep better at night and stay awake better during the day, it's time to put the tips and tricks into practice and get the best sleep you've ever had!

Finally, if you enjoyed this book, please take the time to share your thoughts and post a review on Amazon. It'd be greatly appreciated!

Thank you and good luck!

Made in the USA
Middletown, DE
22 March 2022

63067445R00056